PATRICK LEIGH
FERMOR

LOOSE AS THE WIND

PENGUIN BOOKS

PENGUIN BOOKS

Published by the Penguin Group. Penguin Books Ltd, 27 Wrights Lane, London
w8 5TZ, England. Penguin Books USA Inc., 375 Hudson Street, New York,
New York 10014, USA. Penguin Books Australia Ltd, Ringwood, Victoria, Australia.
Penguin Books Canada Ltd, 10 Alcorn Avenue, Toronto, Ontario, Canada M4V 3B2.
Penguin Books (NZ) Ltd, 182–190 Wairau Road, Auckland 10, New Zealand · Penguin
Books Ltd, Registered Offices: Harmondsworth, Middlesex, England · These
extracts are from *A Time of Gifts* by Patrick Leigh Fermor, published in Penguin
Books 1979. This edition published 1996. Copyright © Patrick Leigh Fermor, 1977.
All rights reserved · Typeset by Rowland Phototypesetting Ltd, Bury St Edmunds,
Suffolk · Printed in England by Clays Ltd, St Ives plc · Except in the United States
of America, this book is sold subject to the condition that it shall not, by way of trade
or otherwise, be lent, re-sold, hired out, or otherwise circulated without the publisher's
prior consent in any form of binding or cover other than that in which it is published
and without a similar condition including this condition being imposed on the sub-
sequent purchaser · 10 9 8 7 6 5 4 3 2 1

CONTENTS

'A splendid afternoon to set out!', said one of the friends who was seeing me off, peering at the rain and rolling up the window.

The other two agreed. Sheltering under the Curzon Street arch of Shepherd Market, we had found a taxi at last. In Half Moon Street, all collars were up. A thousand glistening umbrellas were tilted over a thousand bowler hats in Piccadilly; the Jermyn Street shops, distorted by streaming water, had become a submarine arcade; and the clubmen of Pall Mall, with china tea and anchovy toast in mind, were scuttling for sanctuary up the steps of their clubs. Blown askew, the Trafalgar Square fountains twirled like mops, and our taxi, delayed by a horde of Charing Cross commuters reeling and stampeding under a cloudburst, crept into the Strand. The vehicle threaded its way through a flux of traffic. We splashed up Ludgate Hill and the dome of St Paul's sank deeper in its pillared shoulders. The tyres slewed away from the drowning cathedral and a minute later the silhouette of the Monument, descried through veils of rain, seemed so convincingly liquefied out of the perpendicular that the tilting thoroughfare might have been forty fathoms down. The driver, as he swerved wetly into Upper Thames Street, leaned back and said: 'Nice weather for young ducks.'

A smell of fish was there for a moment, then gone. Enjoining haste, the bells of St Magnus the Martyr and St Dunstan-in-the-East were tolling the hour; then sheets of water were rising from our front wheels as the taxi floundered on between the Mint and the Tower of London. Dark complexes of battlements and tree-tops and turrets dimly assembled on one side; then, straight ahead, the pinnacles and the metal parabolas of Tower Bridge were looming. We halted on the bridge just short of the first barbican and the driver indicated the flight of stone steps that descended to Irongate Wharf. We were down them in a moment; and beyond the cobbles and the bollards, with the Dutch tricolour beating damply from her poop and a ragged fan of smoke streaming over the river, the *Stadthouder Willem* rode at anchor. At the end of lengthening fathoms of chain, the swirling tide had lifted her with a sigh almost level with the flagstones: gleaming in the rain, and with full steam-up for departure, she floated in a mewing circus of gulls. Haste and the weather cut short our farewells and our embraces and I sped down the gangway clutching my rucksack and my stick while the others dashed back to the steps – four sodden trouser-legs and two high heels skipping across the puddles – and up them to the waiting taxi; and half a minute later there they were, high overhead on the balustrade of the bridge, craning and waving from the cast-iron quatrefoils. To shield her hair from the rain, the high-heel-wearer had a mackintosh over her head like a
2 coalheaver. I was signalling frantically back as the hawsers

were cast loose and the gangplank shipped. Then they were gone. The anchor-chain clattered through the ports and the vessel turned into the current with a wail of her siren. How strange it seemed, as I took shelter in the little saloon – feeling, suddenly, forlorn; but only for a moment – to be setting off from the heart of London! No beetling cliffs, no Arnoldian crash of pebbles. I might have been leaving for Richmond, or for a supper of shrimps and whitebait at Gravesend, instead of Byzantium. Only the larger ships from the Netherlands berthed at Harwich, the steward said: smaller Dutch craft like th *Stadthouder* always dropped anchor hereabouts: boats from the Zuider Zee had been unloading eels between London Bridge and the Tower since the reign of Queen Elizabeth.

Miraculously, after the pitiless hours of deluge, the rain stopped. Above the drifts of smoke there was a quickly fading glimpse of restless pigeons and a few domes and many steeples and some bone-white Palladian belfries flying rain-washed against a sky of gunmetal and silver and tarnished brass. The girders overhead framed the darkening shape of London Bridge; further up, the teeming water was crossed by the ghosts of Southwark and Blackfriars. Meanwhile St Katherine's Wharf was sliding offstage and upstream, then Execution Dock and Wapping Old Stairs and the Prospect of Whitby and by the time these landmarks were astern of us, the sun was setting fast and the fissures among the western cloudbanks were fading from smoky crimson to violet.

In the gulfs spanned by catwalks between the warehouses, night was assembling too, and the tiers of loading-loopholes yawned like caverns. Slung with chains and cables weighted with shot, hoists jutted on hinges from precipices of warehouse wall and the giant white letters of the wharfingers' names, grimed by a century of soot, were growing less decipherable each second. There was a reek of mud, seaweed, slime, salt, smoke and clinkers and nameless jetsam, and the half-sunk barges and the waterlogged palisades unloosed a universal smell of rotting timber. Was there a whiff of spices? It was too late to say; the ship was drawing away from the shore and gathering speed and the details beyond the wider stretch of water and the convolutions of the gulls were growing blurred. Rotherhithe, Millwall, Limehouse Reach, the West India Docks, Deptford and the Isle of Dogs were rushing upstream in smears of darkness. Chimneys and cranes plumed the banks, but the belfries were thinning out. A chaplet of lights twinkled on a hill. It was Greenwich. The Observatory hung in the dark, and the *Stadthouder* was twanging her way inaudibly through the nought meridian.

The reflected shore lights dropped coils and zigzags into the flood which were thrown into disarray every now and then, by the silhouettes of passing vessels' luminous portholes, the funereal shapes of barges singled out by their port and starboard lights and cutters of the river police smacking from wave to wave as purposefully and as fast as pikes. Once we gave way to a liner that towered out of the water like a festive block of flats; from Hong Kong, said the steward, as she glided by; and the different notes of the sirens boomed up and downstream as though mastodons still haunted the Thames marshes.

A gong tinkled and the steward led me back into the saloon. I was the only passenger. 'We don't get many in December,' he said; 'It's very quiet just now.' When he had cleared away, I took a new and handsomely bound journal out of my rucksack, opened it on the green baize under a pink-shaded lamp and wrote the first entry while the cruets and the wine bottle rattled busily in their stands. Then I went on deck. The lights on either beam had become scarcer but one could pick out the faraway gleam of other vessels and estuary towns which the distance had shrunk to faint constellations. There was a scattering of buoys and the scanned flash of a lighthouse. Sealed away now beyond a score of watery loops, London had vanished and a lurid haze was the only hint of its whereabouts.

I wondered when I would be returning. Excitement ruled out the thought of sleep; it seemed too important a night. (And in many ways, so it proved. The ninth of December, 1933, was just ending and I didn't get back until January 1937 – a whole lifetime later it seemed then – and I felt like Ulysses, 'plein d'usage et de raison', and, for better or for worse, utterly changed by my travels.)

But I must have dozed, in spite of these emotions, for when I woke the only glimmer in sight was our own reflection on the waves. The kingdom had slid away westwards 5 and into the dark. A stiff wind was tearing through the rigging and the mainland of Europe was less than half the night away.

It was still a couple of hours till dawn when we dropped anchor in the Hook of Holland. Snow covered everything and the flakes blew in a slant across the cones of the lamps and confused the glowing discs that spaced out the untrodden quay. I hadn't known that Rotterdam was a few miles inland. I was still the only passenger in the train and this solitary entry, under cover of night and hushed by snow, completed the illusion that I was slipping into Rotterdam, and into Europe, through a secret door.

I wandered about the silent lanes in exultation. The beetling storeys were nearly joining overhead; then the eaves drew away from each other and frozen canals threaded their way through a succession of hump-backed bridges. Snow was piling up on the shoulders of a statue of Erasmus. Trees and masts were dispersed in clumps and the polygonal tiers of an enormous and elaborate gothic belfry soared above the steep roofs. As I was gazing, it slowly tolled five.

The lanes opened on the Boomjes, a long quay lined with trees and capstans, and this in its turn gave on a wide arm of the Maas and an infinity of dim ships. Gulls mewed and wheeled overhead and dipped into the lamplight, scattering their small footprints on the muffled cobblestones and settling in the rigging of the anchored boats in little explosions of snow. The cafés and seamen's taverns which lay back from the quay were all closed except one which showed a promising line of light. A shutter went up and a stout man in clogs opened a glass door, deposited a tabby on the snow and, turning back, began lighting a stove inside. The cat went in again at once; I followed it and the ensuing fried eggs and coffee, ordered by signs, were the best I had ever eaten. I made a second long entry in my journal – it was becoming a passion – and while the landlord polished his glasses and cups and arranged them in glittering ranks, dawn broke, with the snow still coming down against the lightening sky. I put on my greatcoat, slung the rucksack, grasped my stick and headed for the door. The landlord asked where I was going; I said: 'Constantinople.' His brows went up and he signalled to me to wait: then he set out two small glasses and filled them with transparent liquid from a long stone bottle. We clinked them; he emptied his at one gulp and I did the same. With his wishes for godspeed in my ears and an internal bonfire of Bols and a hand smarting from his valedictory shake, I set off. It was the formal start of my journey.

I hadn't gone far before the open door of the Groote Kirk – the cathedral attached to the enormous belfry – beckoned me inside. Filled with dim early morning light, the concavity of grey masonry and whitewash joined in pointed arches high overhead and the floor diminished along the nave in a chessboard of black and white flagstones. So compellingly did the vision tally with a score of half-forgotten Dutch pictures that my mind's eye instantaneously furnished the void with those seventeenth-century groups which should have been sitting or strolling there: burghers with pointed corn-coloured beards – and impious spaniels that refused to stay outside – conferring gravely with their wives and their children, still as chessmen, in black broadcloth and identical honeycomb ruffs under the tremendous hatchmented pillars. Except for this church, the beautiful city was to be bombed to fragments a few years later. I would have lingered, had I known.

In less than an hour I was crunching steadily along the icy ruts of a dyke road and the outskirts of Rotterdam had already vanished in the falling snow. Lifted in the air and lined with willow trees, the road ran dead straight as far as the eye could see, but not so far as it would have in clear weather, for the escorting willows soon became ghostlike in either direction until they dissolved in the surrounding pallor. A wooden-clogged bicyclist would materialize in a peaked cap with circular black ear pads against frostbite, and sometimes his cigar would leave a floating drift from Java or Sumatra on the air long after the smoker had evaporated. I was pleased by my equipment. The rucksack sat with an easy balance and the upturned collar of my second-hand greatcoat, fastened with a semi-detachable flap which I had just discovered, formed a snug tunnel; and with my old cord breeches, their strapping soft after long use, and the grey puttees and the heavy clouted boots, I was impenetrably greaved and jambed and shod; no chink was left for the blast. I was soon thatched with snow and my ears began to tingle, but I was determined never to stoop to those terrible ear pads.

When the snow stopped, the bright morning light laid bare a wonderful flat geometry of canals and polders and willows, and the sails of innumerable mills were turning in a wind that was also keeping all the clouds on the move – and not only clouds and mills; for soon the skaters on the canals, veiled hitherto by the snowfall, were suddenly scattered as a wind-borne portent came whirling out of the distance and tore through their midst like a winged dragon. It was an ice-yacht – a raft on four rubber-tyred wheels under a taut triangle of sail and manned by three reckless boys. It travelled literally with the speed of the wind while one of them hauled on the sail and another steered with a bar. The third flung all his weight on a brake like a shark's jawbone that sent showers of fragments flying. It screamed past with an uproar of shouts as the teeth bit the ice and a noise like the rending of a hundred calico shirts which multiplied to a thousand as the raft made a sharp right-angle turn into a branch-canal. A minute later, it was a faraway speck and the silent landscape, with its Bruegelish skaters circling as slowly as flies along the canals and the polders, seemed tamer after its passing. Snow had covered the landscape with a sparkling layer and the slaty hue of the ice was only becoming visible as the looping arabesques of the skaters laid it bare. Following the white parallelograms the lines of the willows dwindled as insubstantially as trails of vapour. The 9 breeze that impelled those hastening clouds had met no hindrance for a thousand miles and a traveller moving at a footpace along the hog's back of a dyke above the cloud-shadows and the level champaign was filled with intimations of limitless space.

My spirits, already high, steadily rose as I walked. I could scarcely believe that I was really there; alone, that is, on the move, advancing into Europe, surrounded by all this emptiness and change, with a thousand wonders waiting. Because of this, perhaps, the actual doings of the next few days emerge from the general glow in a disjointed and hap-hazard way. I halted at a signpost to eat a hunk of bread with a yellow wedge of cheese sliced from a red cannon ball by a village grocer. One arm of the signpost pointed to Amsterdam and Utrecht, the other to Dordrecht, Breda and Antwerp and I obeyed the latter. The way followed a river with too swift a current for ice to form, and brambles and hazel and rushes grew thick along the banks. Leaning over a bridge I watched a string of barges gliding downstream underneath me in the wake of a stertorous tug bound for Rotterdam, and a little later an island as slender as a weaver's shuttle divided the current amidstream. A floating reed-fringed spinney, it looked like; a small castle with a steeply pitched shingle roof and turrets with conical tops emerged romantically from the mesh of the branches. Belfries of a dizzy height were scattered haphazard across the landscape. They were visible for a very long way, and, in the late afternoon, I singled one of them out for a landmark and a goal.

It was dark when I was close enough to see that the tower, and the town of Dordrecht which gathered at its foot, lay on the other bank of a wide river. I had missed the bridge; but a ferry set me down on the other shore soon after dark. Under the jackdaws of the belfry, a busy amphibian town expanded; it was built of weathered brick and topped by joined gables and crowsteps and snow-laden tiles and fragmented by canals and re-knit by bridges. A multitude of anchored barges loaded with timber formed a flimsy extension of the quays and rocked from end to end when bow-waves from passing vessels stirred them. After supper in a waterfront bar, I fell asleep among the beer mugs and when I woke, I couldn't think where I was. Who were these bargees in peaked caps and jerseys and sea-boots? They were playing a sort of whist in a haze of cheroot-smoke and the dog-eared cards they smacked down were adorned with goblets and swords and staves; the queens wore spiked crowns and the kings and the knaves were slashed and ostrich-plumed like François I and the Emperor Maximilian. My eyes must have closed again, for in the end someone woke me and led me upstairs like a sleep-walker and showed me into a bedroom with a low and slanting ceiling and an eider-down like a giant meringue. I was soon under it. I noticed an oleograph of Queen Wilhelmina at the bed's head and a print of the Synod of Dort at the foot before I blew the candle out.

The clip-clop of clogs on the cobblestones – a puzzling

sound until I looked out of the window – woke me in the morning. The kind old landlady of the place accepted payment for my dinner but none for the room: they had seen I was tired and taken me under their wing. This was the first marvellous instance of a kindness and hospitality that was to occur again and again on these travels.

Except for the snow-covered landscape and the clouds and the tree-bordered flow of the Merwede, the next two days have left little behind them but the names of the towns I slept in. I must have made a late start from Dordrecht: Sliedrecht, my next halting place, is only a few miles on, and Gorinchem, the next after that, is not much more. Some old walls stick in my memory, cobbled streets and a barbican and barges moored along the river, but, clearest of all, the town lock-up. Somebody had told me that humble travellers in Holland could doss down in police stations, and it was true. A constable showed me to a cell without a word, and I slept, rugged up to the ears, on a wooden plank hinged to the wall and secured on two chains under a forest of raffish murals and graffiti. They even gave me a bowl of coffee and quarter of a loaf before I set off. Thank God I had put 'student' in my passport: it was an amulet and an Open Sesame. In European tradition, the word suggested a youthful, needy, and earnest figure, spurred along the highways of the West by a thirst for learning – thus, notwithstanding high spirits and a proneness to dog-Latin drinking songs, a fit candidate for succour.

During these first three days I was never far from a towpath, but so many and confused are the waterways that unconsciously I changed rivers three times: the Noorwede was the first of them, the Merwede followed, then came the Waal; and at Gorinchem the Waal was joined by the Maas. In the morning I could see the great stream of the Maas winding across the plain towards this rendezvous; it had risen in France under the more famous name of Meuse and then flowed across the whole of Belgium; a river only less imposing than the Waal itself, to whose banks I clung for the remainder of my Dutch journey. The Waal is tremendous; no wonder, for it is really the Rhine. 'The Rijn', in Holland, Rembrandt's native stream, is a minor northern branch of the main flow, and it subdivides again and again, loses itself in the delta and finally enters the North Sea through a drainage canal; while the Waal, gorged with Alpine snows and the waters of Lake Constance and the Black Forest and the tribute of a thousand Rhenish streams, rolls seaward in usurped and stately magnificence. Between this tangle of rivers, meanwhile – whose defections and reunions enclosed islands as big as English shires – the geometric despotism of canal and polder and windmill held firm; those turning sails were for drainage, not grinding corn.

All the country I had traversed so far was below sea-level and without this discipline, which everlastingly redressed the balance between solid and liquid, the whole region would have been wild sea, or a brackish waste of flood and fen. 13

When one looked down from a dyke, the infinity of polders and canals and the meanderings of the many streams were plain to the eye; from a lower vantage-point, only the nearest waters were discernible. But, at ground-level, they all vanished. I was sitting and smoking on a millstone by a barn near the old town of Zaltbommel, when I was alerted by the wail of a siren. In the field a quarter of a mile away, between a church and some woods, serenely though invisibly afloat on the hidden Maas, a big white ship a-flutter with pennants was apparently mooing its way across solid meadows under a cloud of gulls.

The Maas advanced and retreated all day long, and towards evening it vanished to the south. Once out of sight, its wide bed climbed the invisible gradients of Brabant and Limburg, bound for a faraway Carolingian hinterland beyond the Ardennes.

Dark fell while I was trudging along a never-ending path beside the Waal. It was lined with skeleton trees; the frozen ice-puddles creaked under my hobnails; and, beyond the branches, the Great Bear and a retinue of winter constellations blazed in a clear cold sky. At last the distant lights of Tiel, poised on the first hill I had seen in Holland, twinkled into being on the other bank. An opportune bridge carried me over and I reached the market-place soon after ten, somnambulant with fatigue after traversing a vast stretch of country. I can't remember under what mountainous eiderdown or in what dank cell I slept the night.

A change came over the country. For the first time, next day, the ground was higher than sea-level and with every step the equipoise of the elements tilted more decisively in favour of dry land. A gentle rolling landscape of water-meadow and ploughland and heath, with the snow melting here and there, stretched away northward through the province of Guelderland and south into Brabant. The roadside calvaries and the twinkle of sanctuary lamps in the churches indicated that I had crossed a religious as well as a carto-graphic contour line. There were farm buildings which elms and chestnut trees and birches snugly encompassed and Hobbema-like avenues of wintry trees which ended at the gates of seemly manor houses – the abodes, I hoped, of mild jonkheers. They were gabled in semicircles and broken right-angles of weathered brick bordered with white stone. Pigeon lofts saddled the scales of the roofs and the breeze kept the gilded weathervanes spinning; and when the leaded windows kindled at lighting-up time, I explored the interiors in my imagination. A deft chiaroscuro illuminated the black and white flagstones; there were massive tables with bulbous legs and Turkey carpets flung over them; convex mirrors dis-torted the reflections; faded wall-charts hung on the walls; globes and harpsichords and inlaid lutes were elegantly scat-tered; and Guelderland squires with pale whiskers – or their wives in tight bonnets and goffered ruffs – lifted needle-thin wine-glasses to judge the colour by the light of the branching and globular brass candelabra which were secured on chains to the beams and the coffered ceilings.

Imaginary interiors . . . No wonder they took shape in painting terms! Ever since those first hours in Rotterdam a three-dimensional Holland had been springing up all round me and expanding into the distance in conformity with another Holland which was already in existence and in every detail complete. For, if there is a foreign landscape familiar to English eyes by proxy, it is this one; by the time they see the original, a hundred mornings and afternoons in museums and picture galleries and country houses have done their work. These confrontations and recognition scenes filled the journey with excitement and delight. The nature of the landscape itself, the colour, the light, the sky, the openness, the expanse and the details of the towns and the villages are leagued together in the weaving of a miraculously consoling and healing spell. Melancholy is exorcized, chaos chased away and wellbeing, alacrity of spirit and a thoughtful calm take their place. In my case, the relationship between familiar landscape and reality led to a further train of thought.

A second kind of scenery – the Italian – is almost as well known in England as the Dutch, and for the same gallery-haunting reasons. How familiar, at one remove, are those piazzas and arcades! The towers and the ribbed cupolas give way to the bridged loops of a river, and the rivers coil into umbered distances between castled hills and walled cities; there are shepherds' hovels and caverns; the fleece of woods succeeds them and the panorama dies away in fluted mountains that are dim or gleaming under skies with no more clouds than a decorative wreath of white vapour. But this scenery is a backcloth, merely, for lily-bearing angels who flutter to earth or play violins and lutes at Nativities; martyrdoms are enacted in front of it, miracles take place, and mystic marriages, scenes of torture, crucifixions, funerals and resurrections; processions wend, rival armies close in a deadlock of striped lances, an ascetic greybeard strikes his breast with a stone or writes at a lectern while a lion slumbers at his feet; a sainted stripling is riddled with crossbow bolts and gloved prelates collapse with upcast eyes and swords embedded across their tonsures. Now, all these transactions strike the eye with a monopolizing impact; for five centuries and more, in many thousands of frames, they have been stealing the scene; and when the strange deeds are absent, recognition is much slower than it is in the Low Countries, where the precedence is reversed. In Holland the landscape is the protagonist, and merely human events – even one so extraordinary as Icarus falling head first in the sea because the wax in his artificial wings has melted – are secondary details: next to Bruegel's ploughed field and trees and sailing ship and ploughman, the falling aeronaut is insignificant. So compelling is the identity of picture and reality that all along my path numberless dawdling afternoons in museums were being summoned back to life and set in motion. Every pace confirmed them. Each scene conjured up its echo. The masts and quays and gables of a river port, the backyard with a besom leaning against a brick wall, the chequer-board floors of churches – there they all were, the entire range of Dutch themes, ending in taverns where I expected to find boors carousing, and found them; and in every case, like magic, the painter's name would simultaneously impinge. The willows, the roofs and the bell-towers, the cows grazing self-consciously in the foreground meadows – there was no need to ask whose easels they were waiting for as they munched.

These vague broodings brought me – somewhere between Tiel and Nijmegen, it must have been – to the foot of one of those vertiginous belfries which are so transparent in the distance and so solid close to. I was inside it and up half a dozen ladders in a minute and gazing down through the cobwebbed louvres. The whole kingdom was revealed. The two great rivers loitered across it with their scatterings of ships and their barge processions and their tributaries. There were the polders and the dykes and the long willow-bordered canals, the heath and arable and pasture dotted with stationary and expectant cattle, windmills and farms and answering belfries, bare rookeries with their wheeling specks just within earshot and a castle or two, half-concealed among a ruffle of woods. The snow had melted here, or fallen more lightly: blue and green and pewter and russet and silver composed the enormous vista of turf and flood and sky. There was a low line of hills to the east, and everywhere the shine of intruding water and even a faint glimmer, far away to the north, of the Zuider Zee. Filled with strange light, the peaceful and harmonious land slid away to infinity under a rush of clouds.

In the bottom chamber, as I left, an octet of clogged bell-ringers was assembling and spitting on their palms before grasping the sallies, and the clangour of their scales and changes, muted to a soft melancholy by the distance, followed me for the next few miles of nightfall and sharpening chill.

It was dark long before I reached the quays of Nijmegen. Then, for the first time for days, I found myself walking up a slant and down again. Lanes of steps climbed from the crowding ships along the waterfront; between the lamplight and the dark, tall towers and zig-zag façades impended. The quayside lamps strung themselves into the distance beside the dark flow of the Waal and upstream a great iron bridge sailed northwards and away for miles beyond the river. I had supper and after filling in my journal I searched the waterfront for a sailors' doss-house and ended up in a room over a blacksmith's.

I knew it was my last night in Holland and I was astonished how quickly I had crossed it. My heels might have been winged. I was astonished, too, at the impressive, clear beauty of the country and its variety, the amazing light and the sway of its healing and collusive charm. No wonder it had produced so many painters! And the Dutch themselves? Although we were reciprocally tongue-tied, the contact was not quite as slight as these pages must suggest. On foot, unlike other forms of travel, it is impossible to be out of touch; and our exchanges were enough, during this brief journey, to leave a deposit of liking and admiration which has lasted ever since.

Sleep fell so fast and empty of dreams that when I woke at six next morning the night seemed to have rushed by in a few minutes. It was the blacksmith's hammer just under the floor boards which had roused me. I lay as though in a trance, listening to the stop-gap bounces as they alternated with resonant horseshoe notes on the beak of the anvil and when the rhythmic banging stopped, I could hear panting bellows and the hiss of steam and the fidgeting of enormous hoofs, and soon the smell of singeing horn that rose through the cracks in the floor was followed by fresh clangs and finally by the grate of a rasp. My host was shoeing a great blond carthorse with a mane and tail of tousled flax. He waved when I went into his smithy and mumbled good morning through a mouthful of horsenails.

It was snowing. A signpost pointed over the bridge to Arnhem, but I stuck to the south bank and followed the road for the German border. In a little while it veered away from the river and after a few miles I espied two figures in the distance: short of the frontier, they were the last people I saw in Holland. They turned out to be two nuns of St Vincent de Paul waiting for a country bus. They were shod in clogs, they had black woollen shawls over their shoulders and their blue stuff habits, caught in the middle, billowed in many pleats. Their boxwood rosaries hung in loops and crucifixes were tucked in their belts like daggers.

But their two umbrellas were of no avail – the slanting snow invaded their coifs and piled up in the wide triangular wings.

The officials at the Dutch frontier handed back my passport, duly stamped, and soon I was crossing the last furlongs of No Man's Land, with the German frontier post growing nearer through the turning snow. Black, white and red were painted in spirals round the road barrier and soon I could make out the scarlet flag charged with its white disc and its black swastika. Similar emblems had been flying over the whole of Germany for the last ten months. Beyond it were the snow-laden trees and the first white acres of Westphalia.

Up the Rhine

Nothing remains from that first day in Germany but a confused memory of woods and snow and sparse villages in the dim Westphalian landscape and pale sunbeams dulled by clouds. The first landmark is the town of Goch, which I reached by nightfall; and here, in a little tobacconist's shop, the mist begins to clear. Buying cigarettes went without a hitch, but when the shopkeeper said: 'Wollen Sie einen Stocknagel?', I was at sea. From a neat row of them in a drawer, he picked a little curved aluminium plaque about an inch long with a view of the town and its name stamped in relief. It cost a pfennig, he said. Taking my stick, he inserted a tack in the hole at each end of the little medallion and nailed it on. Every town in Germany has its own and when I lost the stick a month later, already barnacled with twenty-seven of these plaques, it flashed like a silver wand.

The town was hung with National Socialist flags and the window of an outfitter's shop next door held a display of Party equipment: swastika arm-bands, daggers for the Hitler Youth, blouses for Hitler Maidens and brown shirts for grown-up SA men; swastika buttonholes were arranged in a pattern which read *Heil Hitler* and an androgynous waxdummy with a pearly smile was dressed up in the full uniform of a *Sturmabteilungsmann*. I could identify the faces in some of the photographs on show; the talk of fellow-gazers revealed the names of the others. 'Look, there's Roehm,' someone said, pointing to the leader of the SA clasping the hand which was to purge him next June, 'shaking hands with the Führer!' Baldur von Schirach was taking the salute from a parade of *Hitlerjugend*; Goebbels sat at his desk; and Goering appeared in SA costume; in a white uniform; in voluminous leather shorts; nursing a lion cub; in tails and a white tie; and in a fur collar and plumed hunting hat, aiming a sporting gun. But those of Hitler as a bare-headed Brownshirt, or in a belted mackintosh or a double-breasted uniform and a peaked cap or patting the head of a flaxen-plaited and gap-toothed little girl offering him a bunch of daisies, outnumbered the others. 'Ein sehr schöner Mann!', a woman said. Her companion agreed with a sigh and added that he had wonderful eyes.

The crunch of measured footfalls and the rhythm of a marching song sounded in a side street. Led by a standard-bearer, a column of the SA marched into the square. The song that kept time to their tread, 'Volk, ans Gewehr!'* – often within earshot during the following weeks – was succeeded by the truculent beat of the *Horst Wessel Lied*: once heard, never forgotten; and when it finished, the singers were halted in a three-sided square, and stood at ease. It was dark now and thick snowflakes began falling across the lamplight. The SA men wore breeches and boots and stiff brown ski-caps with the chin-straps lowered like those of motor bicyclists, and belts with a holster and a cross-brace. Their shirts, with a red arm-band on the left sleeve, looked like brown paper; but as they listened to an address by their commander they had a menacing and purposeful look. He stood in the middle of the empty fourth side of the square, and the rasp of his utterance, even robbed of its meaning, struck a chill. Ironic crescendos were spaced out with due pauses for laughter and each clap of laughter preceded a serious and admonitory drop in key. When his peroration had died away the speaker clapped his left hand to his belt buckle, his right arm shot out, and a forest of arms answered him in concert with a three-fold 'Heil!' to his clipped introductory 'Sieg!' They fell out and streamed across the square, beating the snow off their caps and readjusting their chin-straps, while the standard-bearer rolled up his scarlet emblem and loped away with the flag-pole over his shoulder.

I think the inn where I found refuge was called Zum Schwarzen Adler. It was the prototype of so many I fetched up in after the day's march that I must try to reconstruct it.

The opaque spiralling of the leaded panes hid the snowfall and the cars that churned through the slush outside, and a leather curtain on a semi-circular rod over the doorway kept the room snug from cold blasts. The heavy oak tables were set about with benches, hearts and lozenges pierced the chair-backs, a massive china stove soared to the beams overhead, logs were stacked high and sawdust was scattered on the russet tiles. Pewter-lidded beer-mugs paraded along the shelves in ascending height. A framed colour print on the wall showed Frederick the Great, with cocked hat askew, on a restless charger. Bismarck, white-clad in a breastplate under an eagle-topped helmet, beetled baggy-eyed next door; Hindenburg, with hands crossed on sword-hilt, had the torpid solidity of a hippopotamus; and from a fourth frame, Hitler himself fixed us with a scowl of great malignity. Posters with scarlet hearts advertised Kaffee Hag. Clamped in stiff rods, a dozen newspapers hung in a row; and right across the walls were painted jaunty rhymes in bold Gothic black-letter script:

> Wer liebt nicht Wein, Weib und Gesang,
> Der bleibt ein Narr sein Leben lang!*

Beer, caraway seed, beeswax, coffee, pine logs and melting snow combined with the smoke of thick, short cigars in a benign aroma across which every so often the ghost of sauerkraut would float.

I made room between the bretzel stand, the Maggi sauce bottle and my lidded mug on its round eagle-stamped mat and set to work. I was finishing the day's impressions with a dramatic description of the parade when a dozen SA men trooped in and settled at a long table. They looked less fierce

---

*'Who loves not wine, women and song,
Remains a fool his whole life long!'

25

without their horrible caps. One or two, wearing spectacles, might have been clerks or students. After a while they were singing:

> Im Wald, im grünen Walde
> Da steht ein Försterhaus . . .

The words, describing a pretty forester's daughter in the greenwood, bounced along cheerfully and ended in a crashing and sharply syncopated chorus. *Lore, Lore, Lore*, as the song was called, was the rage of Germany that year. It was followed hotfoot by another that was to become equally familiar and obsessive. Like many German songs it described love under the linden trees:

> Darum wink, mein Mädel, wink! wink! wink!*

The line that rhymed with it was 'Sitzt ein kleiner Fink, Fink, Fink'. (It took me weeks to learn that *Fink* was a finch; it was perched on one of those linden boughs.) Thumps accentuated the rhythm; the sound would have resembled a rugger club after a match if the singing had been less good. Later on, the volume dwindled and the thumping died away as the singing became softer and harmonies and descants began to weave more complex patterns. Germany has a rich anthology of regional songs, and these, I think, were dreamy celebrations of the forests and plains of Westphalia, long sighs of homesickness musically transposed. It was charm-

*'So wave, my maiden, wave, wave, wave.'

ing. And the charm made it impossible, at that moment, to connect the singers with organized bullying and the smashing of Jewish shop windows and nocturnal bonfires of books.

The green and intermittently wooded plains of Westphalia unfolded next day with hints of frozen marsh and a hovering threat of more snow. A troop of workmen in Robin Hood caps marched singing down a side lane with their spades martially at the slope: a similar troop, deployed in a row, was digging a turnip field at high speed and almost by numbers. They belonged to the *Arbeitsdienst*, or Labour Corps, a peasant told me. He was shod in those clogs I have always connected with the Dutch; but they were the universal footgear in the German countryside until much further south. (I still remembered a few German phrases I had picked up on winter holidays in Switzerland, so I was never as completely tongue-tied in Germany as I had been in Holland. As I spoke nothing but German during the coming months, these remnants blossomed, quite fast, into an ungrammatical fluency, and it is almost impossible to strike, at any given moment in these pages, the exact degree of my dwindling inarticulacy.)

I halted that evening in the little town of Kevelaer. It is lodged in my memory as a Gothic side-chapel overgrown with *ex votos*. A seventeenth-century image of Our Lady of Kevelaer twinkled in her shrine, splendidly dressed for Advent in purple velvet, stiff with gold lace, heavily crowned and with a many-spiked halo behind a face like a little   27 painted Infanta's. Westphalian pilgrims flocked to her chapel at other seasons and minor miracles abounded. Her likeness stamped my second *Stocknagel* next morning.

One signpost pointed to Kleve, where Anne of Cleves came from, and another to Aachen: if I had realized this was Aix-la-Chapelle, and merely the name of Charlemagne's capital in German, I would have headed there at full speed. As it was, I followed the Cologne road across the plain. Unmemorable and featureless, it flowed away until the fringes of the Ruhr hoisted a distant palisade of industrial chimneys along the horizon and barred the sky with a single massed streamer of smoke.

Germany! . . . I could hardly believe I was there.

For someone born in the second year of World War I, those three syllables were heavily charged. Even as I trudged across it, early subconscious notions, when one first confused Germans with germs and knew that both were bad, still sent up fumes; fumes, moreover, which the ensuing years had expanded into clouds as dark and baleful as the Ruhr smoke along the horizon and still potent enough to unloose over the landscape a mood of – what? Something too evasive to be captured and broken down in a hurry.

I must go back fourteen years, to the first complete event I can remember. I was being led by Margaret, the daughter of the family who were looking after me, across the fields in Northamptonshire in the late afternoon of 18 June 1919. It was Peace Day, and she was twelve, I think, and I was four. In one of the water-meadows, a throng of villagers had assembled round an enormous bonfire all ready for kindling, and on top of it, ready for burning, were dummies of the Kaiser and the Crown Prince. The Kaiser wore a real German spiked-helmet and a cloth mask with huge whiskers; Little Willy was equipped with a cardboard monocle and a busby made of a hearthrug, and both had real German boots. Everyone lay on the grass, singing 'It's a Long, Long Trail A-winding', 'The Only Girl in the World' and 'Keep the Home Fires Burning'; then, 'Good-byee, Don't Cryee', and 'K-K-K-Katie'. We were waiting till it was dark enough to light the bonfire. (An irrelevant remembered detail: when it was almost dark, a man called Thatcher Brown said, 'Half a mo!' and, putting a ladder against the stack, he climbed up and pulled off the boots, leaving tufts of straw bursting out below the knees. There were protestations: 'Too good to waste,' he said.) At last someone set fire to the dry furze at the bottom and up went the flames in a great blaze. Everyone joined hands and danced round it, singing 'Mademoiselle from Armentières' and 'Pack up Your Troubles in Your Old Kitbag'. The whole field was lit up and when the flames reached the two dummies, irregular volleys of bangs and cracks broke out; they must have been stuffed with fireworks. Squibs and stars showered into the night. Everyone clapped and cheered, shouting: 'There goes Kaiser Bill!' For the children there, hoisted on shoulders like me, it was a moment of ecstasy and terror. Lit by the flames, the figures of the halted dancers threw concentric spokes of shadow across the grass. The two dummies above were beginning to collapse like ghostly scarecrows of red ash. Shouting, waving sparklers and throwing fire-crackers, boys were running in and out of the ring of gazers when the delighted shrieks changed to a new key. Screams broke out, then cries for help. Everyone swarmed to a single spot, and looked down. Margaret joined them, then rushed back. She put her hands over my eyes, and we started running. When we were a little way off, she hoisted me piggy-back, saying, *'Don't look back!'* She raced on across the dark fields and between the ricks and over the stiles as fast as she could run. But I did look back for a moment, all the same; the abandoned bonfire lit up the crowd which had assembled under the willows. Everything, somehow, spelt disaster and mishap. When we got home, she rushed upstairs, undressed me and put me into her bed and slipped in, hugging me to her flannel nightdress, sobbing and shuddering and refusing to answer questions. It was only after an endless siege that she told me, days later, what had happened. One of the village boys had been dancing about on the grass with his head back and a Roman candle in his mouth. The firework had slipped through his teeth and down his throat. They rushed him in agony – 'spitting stars', they said – down to the brook. But it was too late . . .

It was a lurid start. A bit later, Margaret took me to watch trucks full of departing German prisoners go by; then to see *The Four Horsemen of the Apocalypse*, which left a confused

impression of exploding shells, bodies on barbed wire, and

a Prussian officers' orgy in a chateau. Much later on, old copies of *Punch* and *Queen Mary's Gift Book* and albums of war-time cartoons abetted the sinister mystique with a new set of stage properties: atrocity stories, farmhouses on fire, French cathedrals in ruins, Zeppelins and the goose-step; uhlans galloping through the autumn woods, Death's Head Hussars, corseted officers with Iron Crosses and fencing slashes, monocles and staccato laughs . . . (How different from our own carefree subalterns in similar illustrations! Fox terriers and Fox's puttees and Anzora hair-cream and Abdullah cigarettes; and Old Bill lighting his pipe under the star-shells!) The German military figures had a certain terrifying glamour, but not the civilians. The bristling pater-familias, his tightly buttoned wife, the priggish spectacled children and the odious dachshund reciting the Hymn of Hate among the sausages and the beer-mugs – nothing relieved the alien strangeness of these visions. Later still the villains of books (when they were not Chinese) were always Germans – spymasters or megalomaniac scientists bent on world domination. (When did these visions replace the early nineteenth-century stereotype of picturesque principalities exclusively populated – except for Prussia – by philosophers and composers and bandsmen and peasants and students drinking and singing in harmony? After the Franco-Prussian War, perhaps.) More recently, *All Quiet on the Western Front* had appeared; tales of night life in Berlin came soon after . . . There was not much else until the Nazis came into power.

How did the Germans seem, now I was in the thick of them?

No nation could live up to so melodramatic an image. Anticlimactically but predictably, I very soon found myself liking them. There is an old tradition in Germany of benevolence to the wandering young: the very humility of my status acted as an Open Sesame to kindness and hospitality. Rather surprisingly to me, being English seemed to help; one was a rare bird and an object of curiosity. But, even if there had been less to like, I would have felt warmly towards them: I was abroad at last, far from my familiar habitat and separated by the sea from the tangles of the past; and all this, combined with the wild and growing exhilaration of the journey, shed a golden radiance.

Even the leaden sky and the dull landscape round Krefeld became a region of mystery and enchantment, though this great industrial city itself only survives as a landmark for a night's shelter. But, at the end of the next day, the evening flush of Düsseldorf meant that I was back on the Rhine! There, once again, flowed the great river flanked by embankments, active with barges and spanned by an enormous modern bridge (called, slightly vexingly, the Skagerrakbrücke, after the Battle of Jutland) and looking no narrower than when we had parted. Great boulevards diminished in perspective on the other shore. There were gardens and a castle and an ornamental lake where a nearly static and enforcedly narcissistic game of swans were reflected in holes that had been chopped for them in the ice; but no black one that I can remember, like Thomas Mann's in the same piece of water.

I asked a policeman where the workhouse was. An hour's walk led to a sparsely lit quarter. Warehouses and the factories and silent yards lay deep under the untrodden snow. I rang a bell and a bearded Franciscan in clogs unbarred a door and led the way to a dormitory lined with palliasses on plank beds and filled with an overpowering fug and a scattering of whispers. A street lamp showed that all the beds round the stove were taken. I pulled off my boots and lay down, smoking in self-defence. I hadn't slept in a room with so many people since leaving school. Some of my contemporaries would still be there, at the end of their last term, snug, at this very moment (I thought as I fell asleep), in their green curtained cubicles, long after their housemaster's rounds and lights out with Bell Harry tolling the hours and the nightwatchman's voice in the precincts announcing a quiet night.

A long stertorous note and a guttural change of pitch from the next bed woke me with a start. The stove had gone out. Snores and groans and sighs were joining in chorus. Though everyone was fast asleep, there were broken sentences and occasional laughs; random explosions broke out. Someone sang a few bars of song and suddenly broke off. Lying in wait in the rafters all the nightmares of the Rhineland had descended on the sleepers.

It was dark in the yard and still snowing when the monk on duty supplied us with axes and saws. We set to work by lamplight on a pile of logs and when they were cut, we filed past a second silent monk and he handed each of us a tin bowl of coffee in exchange for our tools. Another distributed slices of black bread and when the bowls had been handed in, my chopping-mate broke the icicles off the spout of the pump and we worked the handle in turn to slosh the sleep from our faces. The doors were then unbarred.

My chopping-mate was a Saxon from Brunswick and he was heading for Aachen, where, after he had drawn a blank in Cologne, Duisburg, Essen and Düsseldorf and combed the whole of the Ruhr, he hoped to find work in a pins-and-needles factory. 'Gar kein Glück!' he said. He hunched his shoulders into his lumberjack's coat and turned the flaps of his cap down over his ears. A few people were about now, stooping like us against the falling flakes. Snow lay on all the ledges and sills and covered the pavements with a trackless carpet. A tram clanged by with its lights still on, although daylight was beginning and when we reached the heart of the city, the white inviolate gardens and frozen trees expanded round the equestrian statue of an Elector. What about the government, I asked: were they any help? He said, 'Ach, Quatsch!' ('All rot!') and shrugged as though it were all too taxing a theme for our one-sided idiom. He had been in trouble, and he had no hopes of a turn for the better . . . The sky was loosening and lemon-coloured light was dropping through the gaps in the snow clouds as we crossed the Skagerrak Bridge and wails downstream announced that a ship
34 of heavy draught was weighing anchor. At the crossroads

on the other side we lit the last two cigars from a packet I had bought on the *Stadthouder*. He blew out a long cloud and burst out laughing: 'Man wird mich für einen Grafen halten!', he said: 'They'll take me for a Count!' When he'd gone a few paces, he turned and shouted with a wave: 'Gute Reise, Kamerad!' and struck west for Aachen. I headed south and upstream for Cologne.

After a first faraway glimpse, the two famous steeples grew taller and taller as the miles that separated us fell away. At last they commanded the cloudy plain as the spires of a cathedral should, vanishing when the outskirts of the city interposed themselves, and then, as I gazed at the crowding saints of the three Gothic doorways, sailing up into the evening again at close range. Beyond them indoors, although it was already too dark to see the colours of the glass, I knew I was inside the largest Gothic cathedral in Northern Europe. Except for the little constellation of tapers in the shadows of a side chapel, everything was dim. Women knelt interspersed with nuns and the murmured second half of the *Gegrüsset seist Du, Maria* rose in answering chorus to the priest's initial solo; a discreet clatter of beads kept tally of the accumulating prayers. In churches with open spires like Cologne, one could understand how congregations thought their orisons had a better start than prayers under a dome where the syllables might flutter round for hours. With steeples they follow the uprush of lancets and make an immediate break for it.

Tinsel and stars flashed in all the shops and banners saying *Fröhliche Weihnacht!* were suspended across the streets. Clogged villagers and women in fleece-lined rubber boots slipped about the icy pavements with exclamatory greetings and small screams, spilling their armfuls of parcels. The snow heaped up wherever it could and the sharp air and the lights gave the town an authentic Christmas-card feeling. It was the real thing at last! Christmas was only five days away. Renaissance doors pierced walls of ancient brick, upper storeys jutted in salients of carved timber and glass, triangles of crow-steps outlined the steep gables, and eagles and lions and swans swung from convoluted iron brackets along a maze of lanes. As each quarter struck, the saint-encrusted towers challenged each other through the snow and the rivalry of those heavy bells left the air shaking.

Beyond the Cathedral and directly beneath the flying-buttresses of the apse, a street dropped sharply to the quays. Tramp steamers and tugs and barges and fair-sized ships lay at anchor under the spans of the bridges, and cafés and bars were raucous with music. I had been toying with the idea, if I could make the right friends, of cadging a lift on a barge and sailing upstream in style for a bit.

I made friends all right. It was impossible not to. The first place was a haunt of seamen and bargees shod in tall sea-boots rolled down to the knee, with felt linings and thick wooden soles. They were throwing schnapps down their throats at a brisk rate. Each swig was followed by a chaser of beer, and I started doing the same. The girls who drifted in and out were pretty but a rough lot and there was one bulky terror, bursting out of a sailor's jersey and wearing a bargeman's cap askew on a nest of candy-floss hair, called Maggi – which was short for Magda – who greeted every newcomer with a cry of 'Hallo, Bubi!' and a sharp, cunningly twisted and very painful pinch on the cheek. I liked the place, especially after several schnapps, and I was soon firm friends with two beaming bargemen whose Low German speech, even sober, would have been blurred beyond the most expert linguist's grasp. They were called Uli and Peter. 'Don't keep on saying *Sie*,' Uli insisted, with a troubled brow and an unsteadily admonishing forefinger: 'Say *Du*.' This advance from the plural to the greater intimacy of the singular was then celebrated by drinking *Brüderschaft*. Glasses in hand, with our right arms crooked through the other two with the complexity of the three Graces on a Parisian public fountain, we drank in unison. Then we reversed the process with our left arms, preparatory to ending with a triune embrace on both cheeks, a manoeuvre as elaborate as being knighted or invested with the Golden Fleece. The first half of the ceremony went without a hitch, but a loss of balance in the second, while our forearms were still interlocked, landed the three of us in the sawdust in a sottish heap. Later, in the fickle fashion of the very drunk, they lurched away into the night, leaving their newly created brother dancing with a girl who had joined our unsteady group: my hobnail boots could do no more damage to her 37 shiny dancing shoes, I thought, than the seaboots that were clumping all round us. She was very pretty except for two missing front teeth. They had been knocked out in a brawl the week before, she told me.

I woke up in a bargeman's lodging house above a cluster of masts and determined to stay another day in this marvellous town.

It had occurred to me that I might learn German quicker by reading Shakespeare in the famous German translation. The young man in the bookshop spoke some English. Was it *really* so good, I asked him. He was enthusiastic: Schlegel and Tieck's version, he said, was *almost* as good as the original; so I bought *Hamlet, Prinz von Dänemark*, in a paperbound pocket edition. He was so helpful that I asked him if there were any way of travelling up the Rhine by barge. He called a friend into consultation who was more fluent in English: I explained I was a student, travelling to Constantinople on foot with not much money, and that I didn't mind how uncomfortable I was. The newcomer asked: student of what? Well – literature: I wanted to write a book. '*So!* You are travelling about Europe like Childe Harold?' he said. 'Yes, *yes*! Absolutely like Childe Harold!' Where was I staying? I told them. 'Pfui!' They were horrified, and amused. Both were delightful and, as the upshot of all this, I was asked to stay with one of them. We were to meet in the evening.

The day passed in exploring churches and picture galleries and looking at old buildings, with a borrowed guidebook.

Hans, who was my host, had been a fellow-student at Cologne University with Karl, the bookseller. He told me at dinner that he had fixed up a free lift for me next day on a string of barges heading upstream, all the way to the Black Forest if I wanted. We drank delicious Rhine wine and talked about English literature. The key figures in Germany I gathered, were Shakespeare, Byron, Poe, Galsworthy, Wilde, Maugham, Virginia Woolf, Charles Morgan and, very recently, Rosamond Lehmann. What about Priestley, they asked: *The Good Companions*? And *The Story of San Michele*?

It was my first venture inside a German house. The interior was composed of Victorian furniture, bobbled curtains, a stove with green china tiles and many books with characteristic German bindings. Hans's cheerful landlady, who was the widow of a don at the University, joined us over tea with brandy in it. I answered many earnest questions about England: how lucky and enviable I was, they said, to belong to that fortunate kingdom where all was so just and sensible! The allied occupation of the Rhineland had come to an end less than ten years before, and the British, she said, had left an excellent impression. The life she described revolved round football, boxing matches, fox-hunts and theatricals. The Tommies got drunk, of course, and boxed each other in the street – she lifted her hands in the posture of squaring up – but they scarcely ever set about 39 the locals. As for the colonel who had been billeted on her for years, with his pipe and his fox terriers – what a gentleman! What kindness and tact and humour! 'Ein Gentleman durch und durch!' And his soldier servant – an angel! – had married a German girl. This idyllic world of cheery Tommies and Colonel Brambles sounded almost too good to be true and I basked vicariously in their lustre. But the French, they all agreed, were a different story. There had, it seems, been much friction, bloodshed even, and the ill-feeling still lingered. It sprang mainly from the presence of Senegalese units among the occupying troops; their inclusion had been interpreted as an act of calculated vengeance. The collapse of the Reichsmark was touched on, and Reparations; Hitler cropped up. The professor's widow couldn't bear him: such a mean face! 'So ein gemeines Gesicht!' And that voice! Both the others were against him too, and the whole Nazi movement: it was no solution to Germany's problems; and wrong . . . the conversation slid into a trough of depression. (I divined that it was a theme of constant discussion and that they were all against it, but in different ways and for different reasons. It was a time when friendships and families were breaking up all over Germany.) The conversation revived over German literature: apart from Remarque, the only German book I had read was a translation of *Zarathustra*. Neither of them cared much for Nietzsche, 'But he understood us Germans,' Hans said in an ambiguous tone. The Erasmian pronunciation of Latin

cropped up, followed by the reciting of rival passages from

the ancient tongues: innocent showing off all round with no time for any of us to run dry. We grew excited and noisy, and our hostess was delighted. How her husband would have enjoyed it! The evening ended with a third round of handshakes. (The first had taken place on arrival and the second at the beginning of dinner, when the word *Mahlzeit* was ritually pronounced. German days are scanned by a number of such formalities.)

The evening ended for me with the crowning delight of a bath, the first since London. I wondered if the tall copper boiler had been covertly lit as a result of a lively account of my potentially verminous night in the workhouse . . . 'My husband's study,' my hostess had said with a sigh, when she showed me my room. And here, under another of those giant meringue eiderdowns, I lay at last between clean sheets on an enormous leather sofa with a shaded light beside me beneath row upon row of Greek and Latin classics. The works of Lessing, Mommsen, Kant, Ranke, Niebuhr and Gregorovius soared to a ceiling decoratively stencilled with sphinxes and muses. There were plaster busts of Pericles and Cicero, a Victorian view of the Bay of Naples behind a massive desk and round the walls, faded and enlarged, in clearings among the volumes, huge photographs of Paestum, Syracuse, Agrigento, Selinunte and Segesta. I began to understand that German middle-class life held charms that I had never heard of.

The gables of the Rhine quays were gliding past and, as we gathered speed and sailed under one of the spans of the first bridge, the lamps of Cologne all went on simultaneously. In a flash the fading city soared out of the dark and expanded in a geometrical infinity of electric bulbs. Diminishing skeletons of yellow dots leaped into being along the banks and joined hands across the flood in a sequence of lamp-strung bridges. Cologne was sliding astern. The spires were the last of the city to survive and as they too began to dwindle, a dark red sun dropped through bars of amber into a vague *Abendland* that rolled glimmering away towards the Ardennes. I watched the twilight scene from the bows of the leading barge. The new plaque on my stick commemorated the three Magi – their bones had been brought back from the crusade by Frederick Barbarossa – and the legend of St Ursula and her suite of eleven thousand virgins.

The barges were carrying a cargo of cement to Karlsruhe, where they were due to take on timber from the Black Forest and sail downstream again, possibly to Holland. The barges were pretty low in the water already: the cement sacks were lashed under tarpaulin lest a downpour should turn the cargo to stone. Near the stern of the leading barge the funnel puffed out a rank volume of diesel smoke, and, just aft of this hazard swung the brightly painted and beam-like tiller.

The crew were my pals from the bar! I had been the first to realize it. The others grasped the fact more slowly, with anguished cries of recognition as everything gradually and painfully came back to them. Four untidy bunks lined the walls of the cabin and a brazier stood in the middle. Postcards of Anny Ondra, Lilian Harvey, Brigitte Helm and Marlene Dietrich were pinned on the planks of this den; there was Max Schmeling with the gloves up in a bruising crouch, and two chimpanzees astride a giraffe. Uli and Peter and the diesel engineer were all from Hamburg. We sat on the lower bunks and ate fried potatoes mixed with *Speck*: cold lumps of pork fat which struck me as the worst thing I had ever eaten. I contributed a garlic sausage and a bottle of schnapps – leaving presents from Cologne – and at the sight of the bottle, Uli howled like a beagle in pain. Cologne had been a testing time for them all; they were at grips with a group hangover; but the bottle was soon empty all the same. Afterwards Peter brought out a very elaborate mouth-organ. We sang *Stille Nacht*, and I learnt the words of *Lore, Lore, Lore* and *Muss i denn, muss i denn zum Städtele 'naus*; they said this had been the wartime equivalent of *Tipperary*; then came a Hamburg song about 'Sankt Pauli und die Reeperbahn'. By pulling down a lock of his hair and holding the end of a pocket comb under his nose to simulate a tooth-brush moustache, Uli gave an imitation of Hitler making a speech.

It was a brilliant starry night but very cold and they said I would freeze to death on the cement sacks; I had planned to curl up in my sleeping bag and lie gazing at the stars. So I settled in one of the bunks, getting up every now and then to smoke a cigarette with whoever was on duty at the tiller.

Each barge had a port and starboard light. When another string of barges came downstream, both flotillas signalled with lanterns and the two long Indian files would slide past each other, rocking for a minute or two in each other's wakes. At one point we passed a tug trailing nine barges, each of them twice the length of ours; and later on, the bright speck of a steamer twinkled in the distance. It expanded as it advanced until it towered high above us, and then dwindled and vanished. Deep quarries were scooped out of the banks between the starlit villages that floated downstream. There was a faint glimmer of towns and villages across the plain. Even travelling against the current, we were moving more slowly than we should; the engineer didn't like the sound of the engine: if it broke down altogether, our little procession would start floating chaotically backwards and downstream. Files of barges were constantly overtaking us. As dawn broke, amid a shaking of heads, we tied up at the quays of Bonn.

The sky was cloudy and the classical buildings, the public gardens and the leafless trees of the town looked dingy against the snow; but I didn't dare to wander far in case we were suddenly ready to start. My companions were more heavily smeared with diesel oil each time I returned; the engine lay dismembered across the deck amid spanners and hacksaws in an increasingly irreparable-looking chaos and at nightfall it seemed beyond redemption. We supped nearby and Uli and Peter and I, leaving the engineer alone with his blow-lamp, trooped off to a Laurel and Hardy film – we'd had our eye on it all day – and rolled about in paroxysms till the curtain came down.

At daybreak, all was well! The engine rang with a brisk new note. The country sped downstream at a great pace and the Siebengebirge and the Siegfried-haunted Drachenfels began to climb into the sparkling morning and the saw-teeth of their peaks shed alternate spokes of shadow and sunlight across the water. We sailed between tree-tufted islands. The Rhine crinkled round us where the current ran faster and the bows of vessels creased the surface with wide arrows and each propeller trailed its own long groove between their expanding lines. Among the little tricolours fluttering from every poop the Dutch red-white-and-blue was almost as frequent as the German black-white-and-red. A few flags showing the same colours as the Dutch, but with the stripes perpendicular instead of horizontal, flew from French vessels of shallow draught from the quays of Strasbourg. The rarest colours of all were the black-yellow-and-red of Belgium. These boats, manned by Walloons from Liège, had joined the great river via the Meuse, just below Gorinchem. (What a long way off the little town seemed now, both in time and distance!) A stiff punctilio ruled all this going and coming. Long before crossing or overtaking each other, the appropriate flags were flourished a prescribed number of times from either vessel; and each exchange was followed by long siren blasts. Note answered note; and these salutations and responses and reciprocally fluttering colours spread a charming atmosphere of ceremony over the watery traffic like the doffing of hats between grandees. Sometimes a *Schleppzug* – a string of barges – lay so heavy under its cargo that the coiling bow-wave hid the vessels in turn as though they were sinking one after the other and then emerging for a few seconds as the wave dropped, only to vanish with the next curl of water; and so all along the line. Seagulls still skimmed and swooped and hovered on beating wings for thrown morsels or alighted on the bulwarks and stood there pensively for a minute or two. I watched all this from a nest among the sacks with a mug of Uli's coffee in one hand and a slice of bread in the other.

How exhilarating to be away from the plain! With every minute that passed the mountains climbed with greater resolution. Bridges linked the little towns from bank to bank and the water scurried round the piers on either side as we threaded upstream. Shuttered for the winter, hotels rose above the town roofs and piers for passenger steamers jutted into the stream. Unfabled as yet, Bad Godesberg slipped past. Castles crumbled on pinnacles. They loomed on their spikes like the turrets of the Green Knight before Sir Gawain; and one of them – so my unfolding river map told me – might have been built by Roland. Charlemagne was associated with the next. Standing among tall trees, the palaces of electors and princes and pleasure-loving archbishops reflected the sunlight from many windows. The castle of the Princes of Wied moved out of the wings, floated to the centre and then drifted slowly off-stage again. Was this where the short-reigned Mpret of Albania grew up? Were any of these castles, I wondered, abodes of those romantic-sounding noblemen, *Rheingrafen* and *Wildgrafen*

– Rhine-Counts or Counts of the Forest, or the Wilderness or of Deer? If I had had to be German, I thought, I wouldn't have minded being a Wildgrave; or a Rhinegrave ... A shout from the cabin broke into these thoughts: Uli handed up a tin plate of delicious baked beans garnished with some more frightful *Speck*, which was quickly hidden and sent to join the Rheingold when no one was looking.

On the concertina-folds of my map these annotated shores resembled a historical traffic block. We were chugging along Caesar's *limes* with the Franks. 'Caesar threw a bridge across the Rhine ...' Yes, but where? Later emperors moved the frontier eastward into the mountains far beyond the left bank, where, so they said, the Hercynian forest, home of unicorns, was too dense for a cohort to deploy, let alone a legion. (Look what happened to the legions of Quintilius Varus a hundred miles north-east! Those were vague regions, utterly unlike the shores of the brilliant Rhine: the *Frigund* of German myth, a thicket that still continued after sixty days of travel and the haunt, when the unicorns trotted away into fable, of wolves and elks and reindeers and the aurochs. The Dark Ages, when they reached them, found no lights to extinguish, for none had ever shone there.) Westward the map indicated the outlines of Lothair's kingdom after the Carolingian break-up. Later fragmentations were illustrated heraldically by a jostle of crossed swords and crosiers and shields with closed crowns and coronets and mitres on top, and electoral caps turned up with ermine. Sometimes the hats of cardinals were levitated above their 47 twin pyramids of tassels and an unwieldy growth of crests sprang from the helmets of robber knights. Each of these emblems symbolized a piece in a jigsaw of minute but hardy sovereign fiefs that had owed homage only to the Holy Roman Emperor; each of them exacted toll from the wretched ships that sailed under their battlements; and when Napoleon's advance exorcized the lingering ghost of the realm of Charlemagne, they survived, and still survive, in a confetti of mediatizations. On the terrace of one water-side schloss a strolling descendant in a Norfolk jacket was lighting his mid-morning cigar.

The amazing procession went on all day.

The walled town of Andernach was bearing down on us. The engineer snored in his bunk, Peter was smoking at the tiller and I lolled in the sun on the cabin roof while Uli sent flourishes and grace-notes cascading from his mouth-organ. Two or three bridges and half a dozen castles later, after a final hour or so of snow-covered slopes, we were losing speed under the lee of the Ehrenbreitstein. This colossal and extremely business-like modern fort was a cliff of masonry bristling with casemates and slotted with gun embrasures. The town of Coblenz rose from the other shore with a noble sweep.

We slanted in towards the quay on the west bank; gradually, to prevent the barges bumping into each other or piling up as we lost speed. The whole manoeuvre was for my sake as the others had to hasten on. It was a sad parting: 'Du kommst nicht mit?' they cried. When we were going slow enough, and close enough to the embankment, I jumped ashore. We waved to each other as they steered amidstream again, and Uli unloosed a succession of piercing shrieks from the siren and then a long blast of valediction that echoed amazingly along the cliffs of Coblenz. Then they straightened out and slid under a bridge of boats and sped south.

A point like a flat-iron jutted into the river and a plinth on its tip lifted a colossal bronze statue of Kaiser Wilhelm I many yards into the air among the sparrows and the gulls. This projection of rock and masonry had once been an isolated southern settlement of the Teutonic Knights – to my surprise: I had always imagined these warriors hacking away at Muscovites in a non-stop snowstorm on the shores of the Baltic or the Masurian lakes. The Thirty Years War raged through the place. Metternich was born a few doors away. But a hoarier, more cosmic chronology had singled it out. Two great rivers, rushing blind down their converging canyons, collide under the tip of the flat-iron and the tangled flux of the current ruffles and dwindles downstream till the Rhine's great silted volume subdues the clearer flow of the newcomer. The Moselle! I knew that this loop of water, swerving under its bridges and out of sight, was the last stretch of a long valley of the utmost significance and beauty. A seagull, flying upstream, would look down for scores of miles on tiered and winding vineyards, and swoop, if he chose, through the great black Roman gates of Trier and then over the amphitheatre and across the frontier into Lorraine. Skimming through the weathervanes of the old Merovingian city of Metz, he would settle among the rocks of the Vosges where the stream begins. I was tempted, for a moment, to follow it: but its path pointed due west; I'd never get to Constantinople that way. Ausonius, if I had read him then, might have tipped the scales.

Coblenz is on a slant. Every street tilted and I was always looking across towers and chimney-pots and down on the two corridors of mountain that conducted the streams to their meeting. It was a buoyant place under a clear sky, everything in the air whispered that the plains were far behind and the sunlight sent a flicker and a flash of reflections glancing up from the snow; and two more invisible lines had been crossed and important ones: the accent had changed and wine cellars had taken the place of beer halls. Instead of those grey mastodonic mugs, wine glasses glittered on the oak. (It was under a vista of old casks in a *Weinstube* that I settled with my diary till bedtime.) The plain bowls of these wine glasses were poised on slender glass stalks, or on diminishing pagodas of little globes, and both kinds of stem were coloured: a deep green for Mosel and, for Rhenish, a brown smoky gold that was almost amber. When horny hands lifted them, each flashed forth its coloured message in the lamplight. It is impossible, drinking by the glass in those charmingly named inns and wine cellars, not to drink too much. Deceptively and treacherously, those innocent-looking goblets hold nearly half a bottle and simply by sipping one could explore the two great rivers below and the Danube and all Swabia, and Franconia too by proxy, and the vales of Imhof and the faraway slopes of Würzburg; journeying in time from year to year, with draughts as cool as a deep well, limpidly varying from dark gold to pale silver and smelling of glades and meadows and flowers. Gothic inscriptions still flaunted across the walls, but they were harmless here, and free of the gloom imposed by those boisterous and pace-forcing black-letter hortations in the beer halls of the north. And the style was better: less emphatic, more lucid and laconic; and both consoling and profound in content; or so it seemed as the hours passed. *Glaub, was wahr ist, enjoined a message across an antlered wall, Lieb, was rar ist, Trink, was klar ist.** I only realized as I stumbled to bed how pliantly I had obeyed.

It was the shortest day of the year and signs of the season were becoming hourly more marked. Every other person in the streets was heading for home with a tall and newly felled fir sapling across his shoulder, and it was under a mesh of Christmas decorations that I was sucked into the Liebfrauenkirche next day. The romanesque nave was packed and an anthem of great choral splendour rose from the gothic choir stalls, while the cauliflowering incense followed the plainsong across the slopes of the sunbeams. A Dominican in horn-rimmed spectacles delivered a vigorous sermon. A number of Brownshirts – I'd forgotten all about

*'Believe what is true; love what is rare; drink what is clear.' 51

them for the moment – was scattered among the congregation, with eyes lowered and their caps in their hands. They looked rather odd. They should have been out in the forest, dancing round Odin and Thor, or Loki perhaps.

Coblenz and its great fortress dropped behind and the mountains took another pace forward. Serried vineyards now covered the banks of the river, climbing as high as they could find a foothold. Carefully buttressed with masonry, shelf rose on shelf in fluid and looping sweeps. Pruned to the bone, the dark vine-shoots stuck out of the snow in rows of skeleton fists which shrank to quincunxes of black commas along the snow-covered contour lines of the vineyards as they climbed, until the steep waves of salients and re-entrants faltered at last and expired overhead among the wild bare rocks. On the mountains that overhung these flowing ledges, scarcely a peak had been left without a castle. At Stolzenfels, where I stopped for something to eat, a neo-Gothic keep climbed into the sky on a staircase of vineyards, and another castle echoed it from Oberlahnstein on the other shore. Then another rose up, and another, and yet another: ruin on ruin, and vineyard on vineyard . . . They seemed to revolve as they moved downstream, and then to impend. Finally a loop of the river would carry them away until the dimness of the evening blurred them all and the lights of the shore began to twinkle among their darkening reflections. Soon after dark, I halted at Boppard. It was lodged a little way up the mountain-side so that next morning a fresh length of the river uncoiled southward while the Sunday morning bells were answering our own chimes upstream and down.

When the cliffs above were too steep for snow, spinneys frilled the ledges of shale, and fans of brushwood split the sunbeams into an infinity of threads. Higher still, the gap-toothed and unfailing towers – choked with trees and lashed together with ivy – thrust angles into the air which followed up the impulse of the crags on which they were perched; and, most fittingly, their names all ended in the German word for 'angle' or 'rock' or 'crag' or 'keep': Hoheneck, Reichenstein, Stolzenfels, Falkenburg . . . Each turn of the river brought into view a new set of stage wings and sometimes a troop of islands which the perpetual rush of the river had worn thin and moulded into the swerve of the current. They seemed to float there under a tangle of bare twigs and a load of monastic or secular ruins. A few of these eyots were sockets for towers which could bar the river by slinging chains to either bank and holding up ships for toll or loot or ransom. Dark tales abound.

Fragmentary walls, pierced by old gateways, girdled most of the little towns. I halted in many of them for a glass of wine out of one of those goblets with coloured stems with a slice of black bread and butter, sipping and munching by the stove while, every few minutes, my dripping boots shed another slab of hobnail-impacted snow several inches thick. The river, meanwhile, was narrowing fast and the mountains were advancing and tilting more steeply until there was 53 barely space for the road. A huge answering buttress loomed on the other bank and on its summit, helped by the innkeeper's explanation, I could just discern the semblance of the Lorelei who gave the rock its name. The river, after narrowing with such suddenness, sinks to a great depth here and churns perilously enough to give colour to the stories of ships and sailors beckoned to destruction. The siren of a barge unloosed a long echo; and the road, scanned by brief halts, brought me into Bingen at dusk.

The only customer, I unslung my rucksack in a little Gasthof. Standing on chairs, the innkeeper's pretty daughters, who were aged from five to fifteen, were helping their father decorate a Christmas tree; hanging witch-balls, looping tinsel, fixing candles to the branches, and crowning the tip with a wonderful star. They asked me to help and when it was almost done, their father, a tall, thoughtful-looking man, uncorked a slim bottle from the Rüdesheim vineyard just over the river. We drank it together and had nearly finished a second by the time the last touches to the tree were complete. Then the family assembled round it and sang. The candles were the only light and the solemn and charming ceremony was made memorable by the candle-lit faces of the girls – and by their beautiful and clear voices. I was rather surprised that they didn't sing *Stille Nacht*: it had been much in the air the last few days; but it is a Lutheran hymn and I think this bank of the Rhine was mostly Catholic. Two of the carols they sang have stuck in my memory: *O Du Heilige* and *Es ist ein Ros entsprungen*:

both were entrancing, and especially the second, which, they told me, was very old. In the end I went to church with them and stayed the night. When all the inhabitants of Bingen were exchanging greetings with each other outside the church in the small hours, a few flakes began falling. Next morning the household embraced each other, shook hands again and wished everyone a happy Christmas. The smallest of the daughters gave me a tangerine and a packet of cigarettes wrapped beautifully in tinsel and silver paper. I wished I'd had something to hand her, neatly done up in a holly-patterned ribbon – I thought later of my aluminium pencil-case containing a new Venus or Royal Sovereign wound in tissue paper, but too late. The time of gifts.

The Rhine soon takes a sharp turn eastwards, and the walls of the valley recede again. I crossed the river to Rüdesheim, drank a glass of Hock under the famous vineyard and pushed on. The snow lay deep and crisp and even. On the march under the light fall of flakes, I wondered if I had been right to leave Bingen. My kind benefactors had asked me to stay, several times; but they had been expecting relations and, after their hospitality, I felt, in spite of their insistence, that a strange face at their family feast might be too much. So here I was on a sunny Christmas morning, plunging on through a layer of new snow. No vessels were moving on the Rhine, hardly a car passed, nobody was out of doors, and, in the little towns, nothing stirred. Everyone was inside. Feeling lonely and beginning to regret my flight, I wondered what my family and friends were doing, and 55 skinned and ate the tangerine rather pensively. The flung peel, fallen short on the icy margin, became the target for a sudden assembly of Rhine gulls. Watching them swoop, I unpacked and lit one of my Christmas cigarettes, and felt better.

In the inn where I halted at midday – *where was it?* Geisenheim? Winkel? Östrich? Hattenheim? – a long table was splendidly spread for a feast and a lit Christmas tree twinkled at one end. About thirty people were settling down with a lot of jovial noise when some soft-hearted soul must have spotted the solitary figure in the empty bar. Unreluctantly, I was drawn into the feast; and here, in my memory, as the bottles of Johannisberger and Markobrunner mount up, things begin to grow blurred.

A thirsty and boisterous rump at the end of the table was still drinking at sunset. Then came a packed motorcar, a short journey, and a large room full of faces and the Rhine twinkling far below. Perhaps we were in a castle . . . some time later, the scene changes: there is another jaunt, through the dark this time, with the lights multiplying and the snow under the tyres turning to slush; then more faces float to the surface and music and dancing and glasses being filled and emptied and spilled.

I woke up dizzily next morning on someone's sofa. Beyond the lace curtains and some distance below, the snow on either side of the tramlines looked unseasonably mashed and sooty for the feast of Stephen.

ISABEL ALLENDE · *Voices in My Ear*
NICHOLSON BAKER · *Playing Trombone*
LINDSEY BAREHAM · *The Little Book of Big Soups*
KAREN BLIXEN · *From the Ngong Hills*
DIRK BOGARDE · *Coming of Age*
ANTHONY BURGESS · *Childhood*
ANGELA CARTER · *Lizzie Borden*
CARLOS CASTANEDA · *The Sorcerer's Ring of Power*
ELIZABETH DAVID · *Peperonata and Other Italian Dishes*
RICHARD DAWKINS · *The Pocket Watchmaker*
GERALD DURRELL · *The Pageant of Fireflies*
RICHARD ELLMANN · *The Trial of Oscar Wilde*
EPICURUS · *Letter on Happiness*
MARIANNE FAITHFULL · *Year One*
KEITH FLOYD · *Hot and Spicy Floyd*
ALEXANDER FRATER · *Where the Dawn Comes Up Like Thunder*
ESTHER FREUD · *Meeting Bilal*
JOHN KENNETH GALBRAITH · *The Culture of Contentment*
ROB GRANT AND DOUG NAYLOR · *Scenes from the Dwarf*
ROBERT GRAVES · *The Gods of Olympus*
JANE GRIGSON · *Puddings*
SOPHIE GRIGSON · *From Sophie's Table*
KATHARINE HEPBURN · *Little Me*
SUSAN HILL · *The Badness Within Him*
ALAN HOLLINGHURST · *Adventures Underground*
BARRY HUMPHRIES · *Less is More Please*
HOWARD JACOBSON · *Expulsion from Paradise*
P. D. JAMES · *The Girl Who Loved Graveyards*
STEPHEN KING · *Umney's Last Case*
LAO TZU · *Tao Te Ching*
DAVID LEAVITT · *Chips Is Here*

PENGUIN 60s

LAURIE LEE · *To War in Spain*

PATRICK LEIGH FERMOR · *Loose as the Wind*

ELMORE LEONARD · *Trouble at Rindo's Station*

DAVID LODGE · *Surprised by Summer*

BERNARD MAC LAVERTY · *The Miraculous Candidate*

SHENA MACKAY · *Cloud-Cuckoo-Land*

NORMAN MAILER · *The Dressing Room*

PETER MAYLE · *Postcards from Summer*

JAN MORRIS · *Scenes from Havian Life*

BLAKE MORRISON · *Camp Cuba*

VLADIMIR NABOKOV · *Now Remember*

REDMOND O'HANLON · *A River in Borneo*

STEVEN PINKER · *Thinking in Tongues*

CRAIG RAINE · *Private View*

CLAUDIA RODEN · *Ful Medames and Other Vegetarian Dishes*

HELGE RUBINSTEIN · *Chocolate Parfait*

SIMON SCHAMA · *The Taking of the Bastille*

WILL SELF · *The Rock of Crack As Big As the Ritz*

MARK SHAND · *Elephant Tales*

NIGEL SLATER · *30-Minute Suppers*

RICK STEIN · *Fresh from the Sea*

LYTTON STRACHEY · *Florence Nightingale*

PAUL THEROUX · *Slow Trains to Simla*

COLIN THUBRON · *Samarkand*

MARK TULLY · *Beyond Purdah*

LAURENS VAN DER POST · *Merry Christmas, Mr Lawrence*

MARGARET VISSER · *More than Meets the Eye*

GAVIN YOUNG · *Something of Samoa*

and

Thirty Obituaries from Wisden · SELECTED BY MATTHEW ENGEL

READ MORE IN PENGUIN

For complete information about books available from Penguin and how to order them, please write to us at the appropriate address below. Please note that for copyright reasons the selection of books varies from country to country.

IN THE UNITED KINGDOM: Please write to *Dept. EP, Penguin Books Ltd, Bath Road, Harmondsworth, Middlesex UB7 0DA.*

IN THE UNITED STATES: Please write to *Consumer Sales, Penguin USA, P.O. Box 999, Dept. 17109, Bergenfield, New Jersey 07621-0120.* VISA and MasterCard holders call 1-800-253-6476 to order Penguin titles.

IN CANADA: Please write to *Penguin Books Canada Ltd, 10 Alcorn Avenue, Suite 300, Toronto, Ontario M4V 3B2.*

IN AUSTRALIA: Please write to *Penguin Books Australia Ltd, P.O. Box 257, Ringwood, Victoria 3134.*

IN NEW ZEALAND: Please write to *Penguin Books (NZ) Ltd, Private Bag 102902, North Shore Mail Centre, Auckland 10.*

IN INDIA: Please write to *Penguin Books India Pvt Ltd, 706 Eros Apartments, 56 Nehru Place, New Delhi 110 019.*

IN THE NETHERLANDS: Please write to *Penguin Books Netherlands bv, Postbus 3507, NL-1001 AH Amsterdam.*

IN GERMANY: Please write to *Penguin Books Deutschland GmbH, Metzlerstrasse 26, 60594 Frankfurt am Main.*

IN SPAIN: Please write to *Penguin Books S. A., Bravo Murillo 19, 1° B, 28015 Madrid.*

IN ITALY: Please write to *Penguin Italia s.r.l., Via Felice Casati 20, I-20124 Milano.*

IN FRANCE: Please write to *Penguin France S. A., 17 rue Lejeune, F-31000 Toulouse.*

IN JAPAN: Please write to *Penguin Books Japan, Ishikiribashi Building, 2-5-4, Suido, Bunkyo-ku, Tokyo 112.*

IN GREECE: Please write to *Penguin Hellas Ltd, Dimocritou 3, GR-106 71 Athens.*

IN SOUTH AFRICA: Please write to *Longman Penguin Southern Africa (Pty) Ltd, Private Bag X08, Bertsham 2013.*